AROMATHERAPY FOR URINARY TRACT INFECTION (UTI) TREATMENT

DR MIRIAM KINAI

CONTENTS

ACKNOWLEDGMENTS

I would like to express my sincere gratitude to everyone who contributed in one way or another to the development of this publication.

I would especially like to thank http://www.zazzle.com/ChristianArtGifts for their photographs.

1

WHAT IS AROMATHERAPY?

Aromatherapy is the use of essential oils for their healing benefits.

*****

What Are Essential Oils?

The characteristics of essential oils include:

1. Essential oils are essences extracted from plant material. For example lavender essential oil is extracted from the flowering tops of the lavender plant. Rose essential oil is extracted from the rose flower, eucalyptus from the leaves, ginger from the roots, sandalwood from wood, orange from the fruit, celery from the seeds, cinammon from the bark, frankincense from the gum.

Note that, different essential oils can be produced from the same plant.

For example the bitter orange plant Citrus aurantiumn produces orange essential oil from its fruit rind, neroli essential oil from its flowers and petitgrain essential oil from its leaves.

2. Essential oils are highly concentrated substances.

3. Essential oils do not dissolve in water.

4. Essential oils are not greasy.

5. Essential oils mix well with vegetable oils.

6. Essential oils evaporate, are highly volatile and flammable.

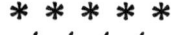

2

CAUTIONARY MEASURES

To get the best results from your use of essential oils and to avoid developing hazardous side effects you should:

1. Always conduct a skin patch test before using a new essential oil.

Do this by applying the essential oil that has been diluted with a carrier oil on the inner aspect of your elbow, bandage it and wait for 24 hours to see if you will develop rashes or itchiness or swelling or any other sign of an allergic reaction.

2. Never apply undiluted essential oils on the skin unless under the supervision of a qualified aromatherapist.

3. Never put essential oils in the eyes. Always close your eyes when inhaling them. If they enter your eyes accidentally, rinse it with copious amounts of water or milk.

4. Never take essential oils internally unless under supervision by a qualified aromatherapist.

5. As ultraviolet light, heat and air can affect essential oils (EOs), store them in tightly shut, dark colored glass bottles in a cool, dark place.

6. Store essential oils away from open flames as they are flammable. Never burn EOs in an oil burner without mixing them with water.

7. The more you open your bottle of essential oils, the more you increase the chances of the oil being oxidized and therefore becoming less effective therapeutically. Therefore, if you buy your essential oils in bulk, decant a small amount into a smaller bottle that you can open daily for regular use.

8. Use your essential oils before they "oxidize" and lose their therapeutic benefits. For example use your citrus oils (orange, lemon, grapefruit, neroli, petitgrain) within one year.

9. Use EOs within 1 month after mixing them with carrier oils.

10. Do not use the same essential oil daily for long periods of time such as 3 months as you may develop sensitivity to it.

11. Do not use essential oils if you are pregnant, have cancer, epilepsy, high blood pressure, liver problems or any other medical condition unless under an aromatherapist's supervision.

Remember that aromatherapy is not supposed to replace conventional medicine. It is supposed to complement it and you should always consult your doctor if you have any medical or mental condition.

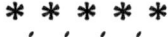

* * * * *

3

CARRIER OILS

Aromatherapy essential oils should first be diluted in water or carrier oils before being applied to the skin because they are very concentrated substances and they may cause severe reactions.

Commonly used carrier oils include Sweet almond oil, Jojoba, Olive oil, Apricot kernel oil, Sunflower oil, Evening primrose oil, Pomegranate oil, Hemp seed oil, Fractionated and Virgin coconut oil.

These carrier oils should be stored in dark glass bottles with tight fitting lids in a cool, dark place.

The choice of a carrier oil or the oil which carries the essential oil to the skin, depends on the therapeutic benefit being sought. Therefore, it is useful to know the different characteristics of the different carrier oils.

***

Sweet Almond Oil

(Prunus amygdalus var. dulcis)

It is one of the most commonly used carrier oils.

It contains vitamins A, B, E, minerals and skin nourishing essential fatty acids.

It has a sweet and nutty aroma.

It is moderately light and has a medium viscosity.

It can be used as a 100% base which means it does not need to be diluted with other carrier oils.

It is an excellent lubricant and is suitable for general massage on normal skin and all other skin types.

It absorbs into the skin moderately quickly leaving a tinge of oil on the skin surface.

It is an excellent moisturizer and thus beneficial for dry skin and mature skin.

It calms sensitive, irritated, inflamed and itchy skin.

It is also beneficial for eczema prone skin.

Do not use it if you have nut allergy.

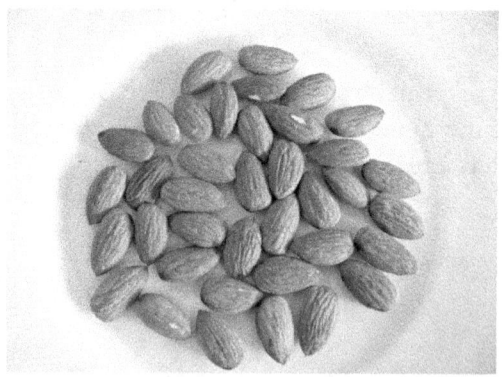

***

Jojoba

(Simmondsia chinensis)

It is a liquid plant wax and not a vegetable oil.

Its chemical composition is similar to that of the skin's own oil or sebum.

It has a very long shelf life since it is highly stable, has a waxy nature and antibacterial properties.

It contains vitamin E, proteins, minerals and skin nourishing fatty acids.

It has a pleasant aroma.

It is moderately light and has a medium viscosity.

It can be used as a 100% base which means it does not need to be diluted with other carrier oils.

It is suitable for general massage on all skin types.

It is readily absorbed by the skin resulting in a non-oily softening effect.

It is especially suitable for use on the face.

It is useful for acne including back acne, due to its antibacterial properties and also because it is non-comedogenic which means that it will not clog the skin pores and contribute to the development of new acne lesions..

It is also beneficial for dry skin, mature skin, oily skin, and conditions with inflamed skin like eczema and psoriasis.

It is useful for arthritis due to its anti-inflammatory properties

It is also useful for hair conditions.

***

Olive Oil

(Olea europaea)

It contains skin nourishing essential fatty acids and natural sunscreens.

It has a cooking olive oil aroma.

It has a thick viscosity.

It is a little thick for massage and is best used when mixed with other carrier oils as a 10-50% additive.

It softens and moisturizes the skin and is thus suitable for dry and inflamed skin.

It is also beneficial for mature or aging skin as well as eczema prone skin.

It has been used to prevent stretch marks during pregnancy.

It is also useful for conditions of the hair and nails.

***

Sunflower oil

(Helianthus annuus)

It has been included here because it is relatively cheap and readily available.

It contains vitamin A, E and skin nourishing essential fatty acids.

It has a sweet, faint aroma

It is light and has a thin viscosity

It is easily absorbed as it penetrates the skin well without leaving an oily feeling on the skin surface after application.

It is suitable for general massage on all skin types.

It softens and moisturizes the skin and is thus suitable for dry skin.

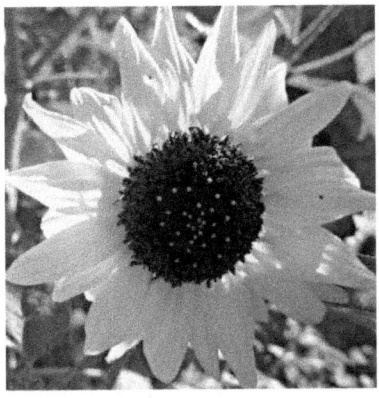

* * * * *

4

UTI ESSENTIAL OILS

Essential oils that are used to treat UTIs include Bergamot, Eucalyptus, Tea tree, German chamomile, Cypress, Juniper berry, Lavender, Cedarwood, Clove, Frankincense and Sandalwood.

BERGAMOT ESSENTIAL OIL

Botanical Name: Citrus bergamia

Method of Extraction: Expressed from fruit peel

Color: Yellowish green

Perfumery Note: Top note

Odor Intensity:

Strength of Initial Aroma: Medium

Aromatic Description: Citrusy and floral

***

Bergamot Essential Oil Safety Information

1. Do not expose the skin to sunlight and UV light for 12-24 hours after using it. It makes the skin more sensitive to the UV light and to developing skin cancer.

2. Do not use bergamot essential oil on children.

3. Do not use bergamot essential oil if you are pregnant or breastfeeding.

4. Avoid it if you have sensitive skin as it can irritate the skin.

5. Do not use bergamot if you are taking medications that make the skin more sensitive to sunlight. These include tetracycline, trimethoprim/sulfamethoxazole, amitriptyline, ciprofloxacin, levofloxacin and related drugs.

6. Do not use it alone for more than 2-3 months as it may lead to sensitization.

7. Always buy your essential oils from a reputable vender to ensure you use high quality therapeutic grade essential oils in your blends.

8. Do not confuse essential oils with fragrance oils as the latter are not the natural essences.

***

EUCALYPTUS ESSENTIAL OIL

Botanical Name: Eucalyptus globulus

Method of Extraction: Steam distilled from the leaves

Color: Clear to yellow

Perfumery Note: Top note

Odor Intensity: 8

Strength of Initial Aroma: Strong

Aromatic Description: Fresh, camphoraceous, medicinal

***

Eucalyptus Essential Oil Safety Information

1. Do not ingest it as it can be fatal when taken orally.

2. Do not use it if you have epilepsy.

3. Do not use it if you have high blood pressure.

4. Do not apply it near a baby's nostrils.

5. Do not store it near homeopathic formulas as it may affect them.

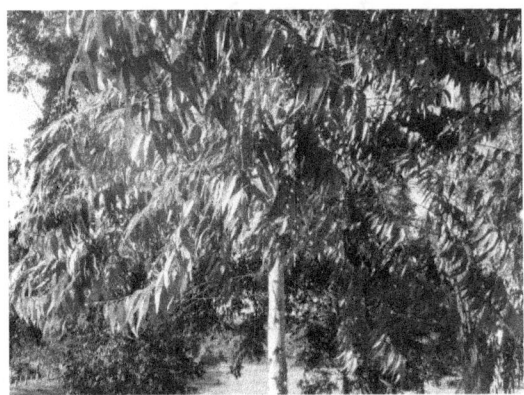

***

LAVENDER ESSENTIAL OIL

Botanical Name: Lavendula officinalis

Method of Extraction: Steam distilled from the flowers

Color: Clear to yellow

Perfumery Note: Middle note

Odor Intensity: 4

Strength of Initial Aroma: Medium

Aromatic Description: Sweet, soothing, floral and fruity

***

Lavender Essential Oil Safety Information

1. Do not use it in pregnancy especially the first 3 months.

2. Do not use it if you are breastfeeding.

3. Do not use it on young children as it may cause breast development in boys (gynaecomastia) and girls (pre-pubescent breast development).

4. Avoid it if you have low blood pressure as you may feel drowsy after using it.

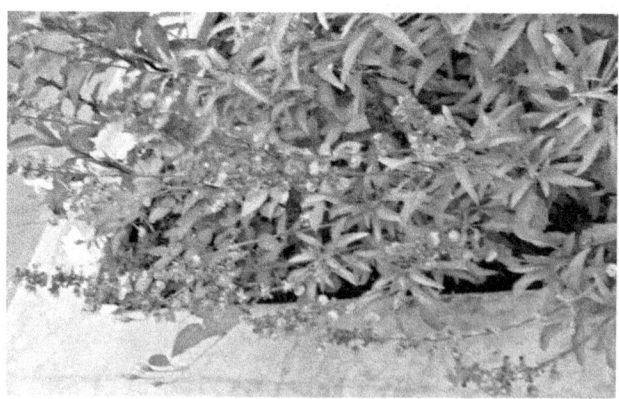

***

SANDALWOOD ESSENTIAL OIL

Botanical Name: Santalum album

Method of Extraction: Steam distilled

Color: Clear to yellow

Perfumery Note: Base note

Odor Intensity: 5

Strength of Initial Aroma: Medium

Aromatic Description: Sweet, woody

Characteristics: Non-toxic, non-irritant, non-photo-toxic

***

Sandalwood Essential Oil Safety Information

1. Avoid using sandalwood if you are allergic to balsams.

2. Do not use it alone for more than 2-3 months as it may lead to sensitization.

3. Always buy your essential oils from a reputable vender to ensure you use high quality therapeutic grade essential oils in your blends.

4. Do not confuse essential oils with fragrance oils as the latter are not the natural essences.

***

TEA TREE ESSENTIAL OIL

Botanical Name: Melaleuca alternifolia

Method of Extraction: Steam distilled

Color: Clear to yellow

Perfumery Note: Top note

Odor Intensity: 7

Strength of Initial Aroma: Strong

Aromatic Description: Fresh, medicinal, camphoraceous

Characteristics: Nontoxic

***

Tea Tree Essential Oil Safety Information

1. It may be irritating on sensitive skins.

2. It may cause sweating when used in high concentrations. Maximum recommended level is 0.1%.

3. Do not use it alone for more than 2-3 months as it may lead to sensitization.

4. Always buy your essential oils from a reputable vender to ensure you use high quality therapeutic grade essential oils in your blends.

5. Do not confuse essential oils with fragrance oils as the latter are not the natural essences.

* * * * *

5

CREATING A
TREATMENT BLEND

The following are the simple four steps you need to take to create a customized essential oil blend for treating urinary tract infections:

1.

Pick the Therapeutic Essential Oils

The first step is to pick the essential oils that can treat your condition.

Therefore if you want to treat a UTI the essential oils that you can use include Bergamot, Eucalyptus, Tea tree, German chamomile, Cypress, Juniper berry, Lavender, Cedarwood, Clove, Frankincense and Sandalwood.

***

2.

Check the Safety Precautions

The second step is to check the contraindications or safety information for each of the essential oils that can be used to treat your condition to make sure that you can use them. For example,

If you are pregnant or breastfeeding do not use/avoid the following:

Essential oils: Angelica, Basil, Bergamot, Black Pepper, Carrot Seed, Cedarwood, Cinnamon Leaf, Clary Sage, Cypress, Fennel, Frankincense, Geranium, Jasmine, Juniper, Lavender, Lemongrass, Marjoram Sweet, Myrrh, Niaouli, Peppermint, Roman Chamomile, Rosemary, Thyme, Yarrow

Carrier oils: Calendula, Castor

Do not use/avoid the following in young children:

Essential oils: Bergamot, Eucalyptus, Lavender, Lemongrass, Niaouli, Peppermint, Rose, Rosemary, Yarrow

If you are trying to conceive do not use/avoid the following:

Carrier oils: Calendula

If you are having your menstrual periods do not use/avoid the following:

Carrier oils: Castor

If you have sensitive skin do not use/avoid the following:

Essential oils: Basil, Bergamot, Black Pepper, Fennel, Lemon, Lemongrass, Nutmeg, Orange, Peppermint, Tea Tree, Ylang Ylang

If you have epilepsy do not use/avoid the following:

Essential Oils: Eucalyptus, Fennel, Peppermint, Rosemary

AROMATHERAPY FOR URINARY TRACT INFECTION (UTI) TREATMENT

If you have high blood pressure do not use/avoid the following:

Essential oils: Eucalyptus, Peppermint, Rosemary, Thyme

If you have low blood pressure do not use/avoid the following:

Essential oils: Lavender, Lemon, Marjoram, Ylang Ylang

If you have kidney or liver disease do not use/avoid the following:

Essential oils: Black Pepper

If you have insomnia or sleeplessness do not use/avoid the following:

Essential oils: Peppermint, Rosemary

If you have irregular heart beat or cardiac fibrillation do not use/avoid the following:

Essential oils: Peppermint

If you have endometriosis, ovarian cysts, uterine cysts, breast cancer or you are at high risk for developing breast cancer do not use/avoid the following:

Essential oils: Clary sage

If you have glaucoma do not use/avoid the following:

Essential oils: Lemongrass

If you have prostatic hyperplasia do not use/avoid the following:

Essential oils: Lemongrass

If you have anorexia nervosa do not use/avoid the following:

Essential oils: Patchouli

If you have frequent headaches do not use/avoid the following:

Essential oils: Clary sage

If you have fever do not use/avoid the following:

Essential oils: Rosemary

If you have nerve problems do not use/avoid the following:

Essential oils: Rosemary

If you are allergic to lemons do not use/avoid the following:

Essential oils: Lemon

If you are allergic to nuts do not use/avoid the following:

Carrier oils: Sweet almond oil

If you are allergic to ragweed, chrysanthemums, marigolds, daisies and other plants from the Asteraceae/Compositae family do not use/ avoid the following:

Essential oils: Roman chamomile

Carrier oils: Sunflower Oil, Calendula

If you are allergic to balsams do not use/avoid the following:

Essential oils: Sandalwood, Petitgrain

If you are allergic to perfumes and cosmetics do not use/avoid the following:

Essential oils: Jasmine, Myrrh, Patchouli, Palmarosa

If you are allergic to spicy food do not use/avoid the following:

Essential oils: Jasmine, Patchouli

If you are taking medications that make the skin more sensitive to sunlight like tetracycline, trimethoprim/sulfamethoxazole, amitriptyline, ciprofloxacin, levofloxacin, etc do not use/avoid the following:

Essential oils: Grapefruit, Lemon, Lemongrass, Orange, Bergamot, Peppermint

AROMATHERAPY FOR URINARY TRACT INFECTION (UTI) TREATMENT

If you are taking sedatives, high blood pressure and diabetes medications do not use/avoid the following:

Carrier oils: Calendula

If you will be exposing your skin to sunlight or UV radiation or using a sun bed or sunbathing in the next 12-24 hours do not use/avoid the following:

Essential oils: Angelica, Cedarwood, Grapefruit, Lemon, Lemongrass, Orange, Bergamot, Grapefruit, Peppermint

If you will be driving or operating machines do not use/avoid the following:

Essential oils: Clary sage

If you will be drinking alcohol do not use/avoid the following:

Essential oils: Clary sage

***

3.

Choose the Scents you Love

The third step is to pick the essential oils with the scents that you love from those that you can safely use.

Therefore, if you love:

Fresh scents use lemon, orange, bergamot, rosemary, peppermint

Floral scents use rose, lavender, geranium, ylang ylang

Fruity scents use Roman chamomile, clary sage

Spicy scents use clove, marjoram, patchouli

Woody scents use sandalwood, cedar

Medicinal scents use eucalyptus, tea tree

4.

Blend your Chosen Essential Oils

The fourth step is to blend the essential oils you have chosen.

To create well balanced essential oil blends, you have to consider the volatility of the different essential oils and mix the essential oils appropriately. To do this, you have to know whether an essential oil is a top note, a middle note or a base note.

Top Notes

These are the essential oils with scents that evaporate the fastest and therefore they are first ones you smell. These scents are generally light, flowery, fruity and uplifting.

Examples of top notes include bergamot, clary sage, eucalyptus, lemon, orange, petitgrain and tea tree.

***

Middles Notes

These scents do not evaporate as fast as the top notes. They are generally spicy, herbal and balancing.

Examples of middle notes include roman chamomile essential oil, cypress essential oil, geranium essential oil, juniper berry essential oil, lavender essential oil, sweet marjoram essential oil, peppermint essential oil, rosemary essential oil and rosewood essential oil.

***

Base Notes

These scents are the slowest to evaporate and therefore the last ones you smell. They are generally heavy and woodsy.

Examples of base notes include sandalwood and ylang ylang.

***

General Rules of Blending Essential Oils

1. Decide what condition you want your essential oil blend or essential oil recipe to manage.

2. Choose approximately 3 pure, organic essential oils that can manage that condition.

3. Divide those essential oils into top notes, middle notes and base notes.

4. Blend your essential oils by adding 1 drop of the base note for every 2 drops of the middle note and 3 drops of the top note into a dark bottle.

5. Begin by adding the base notes and after adding each essential oil into the bottle, swirl it around and smell it before you add the next essential oil.

6. After getting a scent that pleases you or the number or essential oil drops required for a specific recipe, you can now add the essential oils blend to the other ingredients.

7. These are not fixed aromatherapy rules and you can bend them to create your perfect essential oil blend. For example, you can blend by adding just one drop of each essential oil until you get your desired scent.

8. Always have a notebook at hand to record the number of drops of each essential oil you have added to create that particular blend.

***

Practical Example of Blending Essential Oils

1. Decide what condition you want your essential oil blend to manage.

Urinary tract infection (UTI)

2. Choose approximately three essential oils that can manage that condition.

Lavender essential oil, bergamot essential oil and tea tree essential oil

3. Divide those essential oils into top notes, middle notes and base notes.

Top note: bergamot and tea tree, Middle note: lavender

4. Blend your essential oils by adding 1 drop of the base note for every 2 drops of the middle note and 3 drops of the top note into a dark bottle.

5. Begin by adding the base notes and after adding each essential oil into the bottle, swirl it around and smell it before you add the next essential oil.

b) Add 2 drops of lavender essential oil, swirl and sniff

c) Add 3 drops of bergamot and 3 drops of tea tree eucalyptus essential oil, swirl and sniff

6. After getting a scent that pleases you or the total number of drops you need for a recipe, you can now add the essential oils blend to the other ingredients.

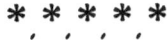

* * * * *

6

AROMATHERAPY UTI TREATMENT RECIPES

The first step in using essential oils is to do a patch test for each of the essential oils that you want to use.

To do this, simply apply the essential oil that has been diluted with a carrier oil on the inner aspect of your elbow, bandage it and wait for 24 hours to see if you will develop rashes or itchiness or swelling or any other sign of an allergic reaction. If you do, do not use that essential oil.

The second step is to create the UTI essential oil blend. You can create a simple one by mixing 20 drops of lavender essential oil, 30 drops of bergamot and 30 drops of tea tree in a dark bottle. We will refer to this mixture as the "UTI Blend" in the recipes.

Therefore, if the recipe says, "Add 12 drops of the UTI Blend", you simply add 12 drops of this mixture of essential oils.

If you just want to buy one aromatherapy oil to experiment with, I would recommend tea tree essential oil. Likewise, if the recipe says, "Add 12 drops of the UTI Blend", you simply add 12 drops of tea tree essential oil.

***

Sitz Bath or Hip Bath.

Add 7 drops of the "UTI Blend" to water in a bowl that is large enough for you to sit in with the water reaching the hip level. Soak in it for 15 minutes. Repeat this twice or thrice a day.

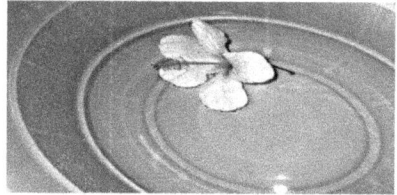

Aromatherapy Bath.

Create a healing bath by dispersing 20 drops of the "UTI Blend" in your warm bath water. You can also mix it with milk to help it disperse.

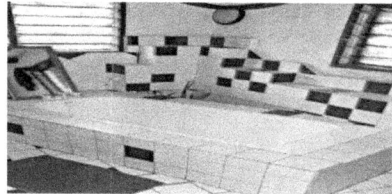

Bath Gel.

Add 50 drops (2.5 ml or ½ teaspoons) of the "UTI Blend" to one cup (8 oz or 250 ml) of unscented bath gel or liquid soap to create a healing bath gel.

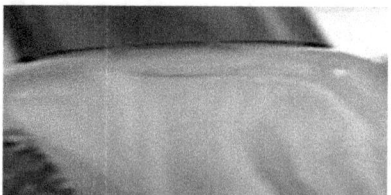

Body Massage Oil.

Add 50 drops (2.5 ml or ½ teaspoons) of the "UTI Blend" to one cup (8 oz or 250 ml) of sweet almond oil or any other carrier oil to create a UTI Treatment Body Massage Oil. Use it to massage your lower abdomen and back.

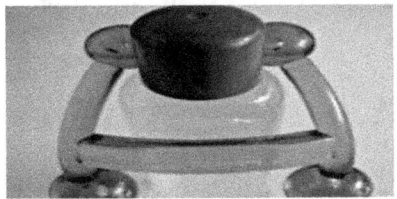

Abdominal Compress.

Add 25 drops (1.25 ml or ¼ teaspoon) of the "UTI Blend" to ½ cup (4 oz or 125 ml) of warm water and mix it, dip a hand towel in it and wring out the excess water. Apply it to your lower abdomen and rest for a few minutes as the healing oils penetrate. Once the towel cools, dip it in the warm water and repeat the process two or three times preferably after massaging the area with the UTI Treatment Body Massage Oil.

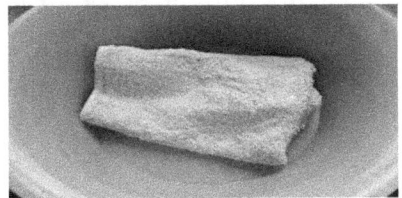

Body Wrap.

Add 20 drops of the "UTI Blend" to 3 oz (100 ml) of distilled water and spray it on a towel. Wrap your lower abdomen and back with the towel and then wrap a plastic sheet around it. Relax for 20 minutes to give the healing oils time to penetrate before unwrapping yourself.

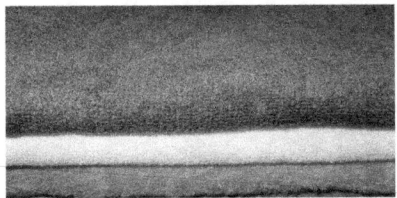

Back Compress.

Add 25 drops (1.25 ml or ¼ teaspoon) of the "UTI Blend" to ½ cup (4 oz or 125 ml) of warm water and mix it, dip a hand towel in it and wring out the excess water. Apply it to your back and rest for a few minutes as the healing oils penetrate. Once the towel cools, dip it in the warm water and repeat the process two or three times preferably after massaging the area with the UTI Treatment Body Massage Oil.

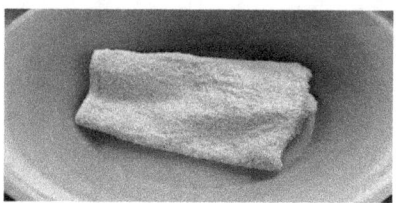

Body Oil.

Add 50 drops (2.5 ml or ½ teaspoons) of an immune boosting essential oil like tea tree, lavender, eucalyptus or bergamot essential oil to one cup (8 oz or 250 ml) of sweet almond oil or any other carrier oil to create a healing. Apply it to your skin after bathing and patting it dry but while it is still moist to lock in the moisture and healing benefits of the essential oil. As you apply it, pay special attention to the pelvis area, back and thighs.

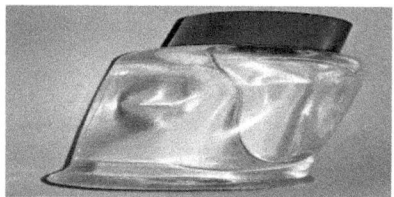

Panty Liner.

Add 6 drops of the "UTI Blend" to your panty liner or pad.

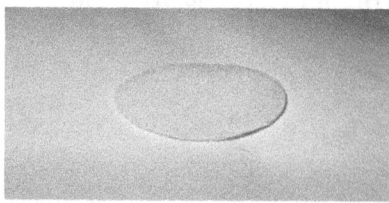

Aloe Vera Aromatherapy Gel.

Add 50 drops of the "UTI Blend" to one cup (8 oz or 250 ml) of natural aloe vera gel to create a non-greasy, healing moisturizer.

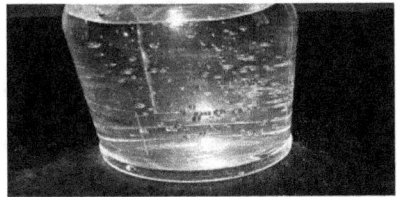

Healing Salve.

Melt 1 oz. (30 grams) of beeswax with 8 oz. (250 ml or 1 cup) of olive oil or any other vegetable oil in a double boiler. Remove from the heat source and one the mixture cools add up to 50 drops (2.5 ml or ½ teaspoon) of the "UTI Blend". Pour the mixture into storage tins and allow it to cool completely. Apply it to your lower abdomen and back.

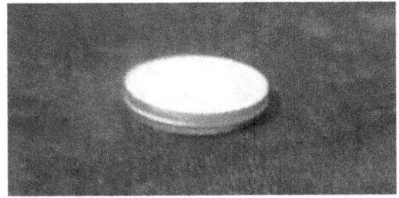

Body Lotion.

Heat 6 oz (190 ml) of sweet almond oil and 1.5 oz (45 grams) of grated beeswax in a double boiler until they mix. Remove from the heat and let the mixture cool completely. Put 8 oz (250 ml) water in a blender and with the blender on high speed, slowly pour in the cooled vegetable oil and beeswax mixture. Blend until the mixture emulsifies or forms a thick lotion. Add 10-20 drops of the "UTI Blend". Pour the lotion in a jar.

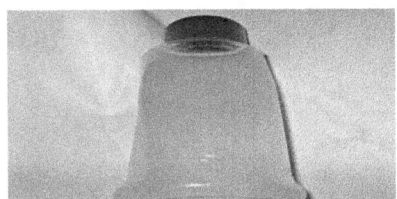

Healing Petroleum Jelly.

Melt 2 teaspoons of a petroleum jelly like Vaseline, add 6 drops of the "UTI Blend" when cool and then pour into a jar.

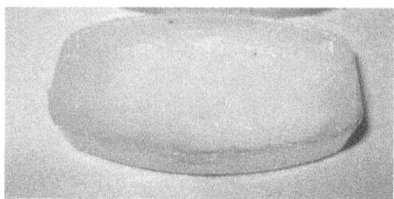

Facial Steamer.

Add 50 drops of an immune boosting essential oil like tea tree, lavender, eucalyptus or bergamot essential oil (or the number or drops recommended by the manufacturer) to one cup (8oz or 250 ml) of water and put it on your facial steamer or sauna.

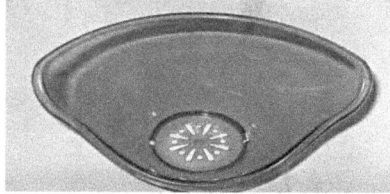

Scent Balls.

Add 6 drops of an immune boosting essential oil like tea tree, lavender, eucalyptus or bergamot essential oil to your handkerchief or a cotton ball and sniff it throughout the day.

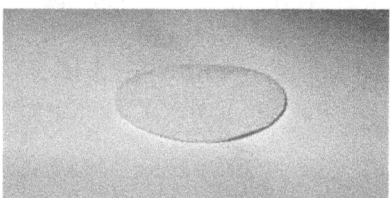

Scented Salts.

Mix 1 cup Epsom salts with 1 cup sea salt and add 50 drops (2.5 ml) of an immune boosting essential oil like tea tree, lavender, eucalyptus or bergamot essential oil in a glass jar with a tight lid. Open the jar and take a whiff of the scent several times during the day.

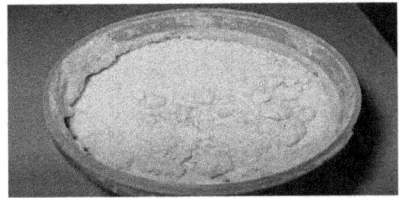

Room Fragrance.

Add 24 drops of an immune boosting essential oil like tea tree, lavender, eucalyptus or bergamot essential oil your diffuser. If your diffuser comes with instructions, use the number of drops recommended by the manufacturer.

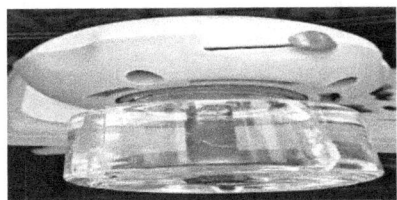

Room Scent.

Add 12 drops of an immune boosting essential oil like tea tree, lavender, eucalyptus or bergamot essential oil ¼ cup (2 oz or 60 ml) of water, place it on an oil warmer and light the candle to scatter the soothing scent.

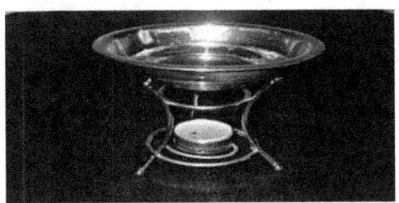

Air Freshener.

Create your own air freshener by adding a total of 250 drops (12.5 ml or 2.5 teaspoons) of an immune boosting essential oil like tea tree, lavender, eucalyptus or bergamot essential oil to one cup (8 oz or 250 ml) of water in a spray bottle and spray it around your room.

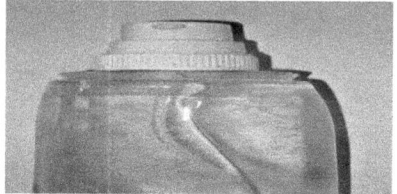

Aroma Ring Scent.

Add 5 drops of an immune boosting essential oil like tea tree, lavender, eucalyptus or bergamot essential oil to an aroma oil ring, place it on top of your lamp bulb, light the lamp and experience relaxing light.

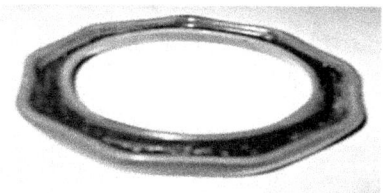

Car Diffuser.

Add an immune boosting essential oil like tea tree, lavender, eucalyptus or bergamot essential oil to your car's diffuser according to the manufacturer's instructions and let the healing scent envelope you as you drive.

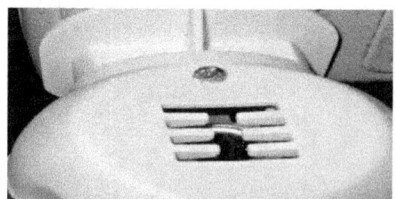

###

ABOUT THE AUTHOR

Dr. Miriam Kinai is a medical doctor and a certified clinical aromatherapy practitioner.

You can visit her blog at http://www.MyBlogBookClub.com or follow her on twitter at http://twitter.com/AlmasiHealth

Email enquiries to almasihealthcare@yahoo.com with BOOKS as your subject.

HERBS AND SPICES FOR THE COOK, HEALER AND BEAUTICIAN

Herbs and Spices for the Cook, Healer and Beautician uses color pictures and clear explanations to teach you about more than 70 healing herbs and spices.

You will learn about their:

* Therapeutic (healing) uses

* Drug interactions

* Contraindications (when not to use them)

* Cooking tips

* Beauty tips

*****

INTERNATIONAL GOURMET HERB AND SPICE BLENDS

International Gourmet Herb and Spice Blends teaches you how to prepare exotic herb and spice blends from around the world. You will discover the recipes for:

* Barbecue Rub, Cajun, Apple Pie and Pumpkin Pie Spice Mixes from America

* Pudding Spice Mix from Britain

* 5 Spice Mix from China

* Berbere Spice Mix from Ethiopia

* Curry Powder and Garam Masala from India

* Bouquet Garni, Herbs de Provence and Quatre Epices from France

* Herb Mix from Italy

* Jerk Seasoning from Jamaica

* Shichimi Togarashi from Japan

* Pilau Spice Blend from Kenya

* Chili Powder from Mexico

* Baharat Spice Blend from the Middle East

* Ras El Hanout from Morocco

*****

THE QUICK GOURMET CHEF

The Quick Gourmet is an essential culinary skills cookbook which teaches how to make simple, divine dishes.

You will learn how to make:

* Hot Chocolate Mixes and Drinks

* Hot Chai Tea Mixes and Drinks

* Hot Coffee Mixes and Drinks

* Sensational Smoothies

* Non-Dairy Smoothies

* Chocolate Covered Strawberries

* Chocolate Truffles

* Healthy Chicken Salads

* Healthy Tuna Salads

* Savory Salsas

* Herb Butter

* Cheese Dips and Sauces

* Gourmet Sandwiches

* Perfect Hard Boiled Eggs

* A Cheese Board

* Natural Food Color

*****

HOW TO STYLE AND PHOTOGRAPH FOOD

Regardless of whether you are an aspiring food blogger or you want to make money online selling stock photos, How To Style and Photograph Food, uses color pictures and clear explanations to teach you the food photography tips that can help you improve your digital camera photography skills so that you can begin photographing food like a pro.

You will learn:

* The equipment that you need

* How to set up the lighting

* How to prepare the stage

* How to style the food

* How to shoot the food

*****

HOW TO MAKE NATURAL SKIN CARE PRODUCTS VOLUME 1

How To Make Natural Skin Care Products Volume 1 by Dr Miriam Kinai is filled with recipes for making organic bath and body products for normal, sensitive, oily and dry skin types as well as therapeutic products to manage mature skin, prematurely aging skin, cellulite, eczema, psoriasis, ringworms, dandruff, thinning hair, menopausal symptoms, pre-menstrual tension (PMS), painful periods, arthritis, stress, sadness or depression, mental exhaustion and insomnia.

This book also teaches you the best vegetable oils, essential oils, natural butters and herbs to use when making products for different skin types physical conditions. You will learn how to make:

* Bath bombs

* Bath melts

* Bath salts

* Bath teas

* Body butters

* Body lotions

* Body scrubs

* Healing balms and body creams

* Herb infused oils

* Natural soap

How to Make Natural Skin Care Products Volume 1 will leave you with a clear understanding of how to make bath and beauty products to use in your home or to give as gifts or to sell and make money.

*****

ORGANIC SKIN CARE PRODUCT INGREDIENTS

Organic Skin Care Product Ingredients teaches you about the different natural substances that can be used to create natural bath and beauty products to use in your home or to give as gifts to your loved ones or to sell and make money.

You will learn about:

* Natural butters

* Natural clays

* Natural colorants

* Natural exfoliants

* Natural fragrances

* Natural oils

* Natural preservatives

*****

THE ESSENTIALS OF AROMATHERAPY ESSENTIAL OILS

The Essentials of Aromatherapy Essential Oils by Dr Miriam Kinai teaches you how to use aromatherapy oils to improve your physical, mental and emotional well being.

The author's experience as a medical doctor and clinical aromatherapy practitioner have enabled her to write a highly informative guide for those who want to utilize the healing benefits of these natural plant essences.

You will discover:

* The safety information and therapeutic uses of 18 essential oils

* How to blend essential oils

* The characteristics and uses of 14 carrier oils

* How to Dilute Essential Oils with Carrier Oils

* How to Use Essential Oils

* Cautionary Measures when using Essential Oils

* Numerous Essential Oil Recipes for bath products as well as skin care and hair care products

The Essentials of Aromatherapy Essential Oils will leave you with a clear understanding of how you can safely use aromatherapy essential oils to heal yourself naturally.

*****

CARRIER OILS GUIDE

Carrier Oils Guide teaches you the characteristics, health benefits and uses of commonly used carrier oils. You will learn about:

* Apricot Kernel Oil

* Avocado Oil

* Borage Seed Oil

* Calendula Oil

* Carrot Seed Oil

* Castor Oil

* Evening Primrose Oil

* Fractionated Coconut Oil

* Jojoba

* Olive Oil

* Rosehip Oil

* Sunflower Oil

* Sweet Almond Oil

* Virgin Coconut Oil

* Useful formulas for Diluting Essential Oils with Carrier Oils

*****

MEDICAL AROMATHERAPY FOR HEALTH PROFESSIONALS

Medical Aromatherapy for Healthcare Professionals by Dr Miriam Kinai teaches you how to use essential oils to treat physical diseases and emotional disorders.

The author's experience as a medical doctor and clinical aromatherapy practitioner have enabled her to write a highly informative guide for those who want to utilize the healing benefits of these natural plant essences.

You will discover how to use essential oils to:

* Treat skin diseases like acne, eczema and psoriasis

* Treat other physical diseases like high blood pressure, arthritis, coughs and colds

* Manage mental and emotional conditions like anxiety, depression, anger and stress

* Relieve the symptoms of menopause and premenstrual tension

* Lessen insomnia and impotence

Medical Aromatherapy for Healthcare Professionals is therefore an essential resource for holistic healthcare practitioners like massage therapists, naturopaths and herbalists.

It is also a useful resource for conventional medicine healthcare providers like physicians and nurses who want to begin practicing integrative medicine and for patients who want to improve their health naturally by using aromatherapy oils.

*****

AROMATHERAPY COURSE

Aromatherapy Course by Dr Miriam Kinai tutors you on how to use essential oils to improve your physical, mental and emotional well being.

The author's experience as a medical doctor and clinical aromatherapy practitioner have enabled her to create a highly informative course on how to use these natural plant essences.

You will learn:

* The safety information and therapeutic uses of essential oils like clary sage, eucalyptus, geranium, grapefruit, lavender, lemon, lemongrass, marjoram, orange (sweet), patchouli, peppermint, Roman chamomile, rose, rosemary, sandalwood, spearmint, tea tree and ylang ylang.

* The safety information and therapeutic uses of carrier oils like apricot kernel oil, avocado oil, borage seed oil, calendula oil, carrot seed oil, castor oil, evening primrose oil, fractionated coconut oil, jojoba, olive oil, rosehip oil, sunflower oil, sweet almond oil and virgin coconut oil.

* How to blend essential oils

* How to dilute essential oils with carrier oils

* How to administer essential oils

* How to make natural healing products from numerous aromatherapy recipes

* How to utilize the healing benefits of essentials oils even if you do not have prior training in aromatherapy

The Aromatherapy Course will leave you with a clear understanding of how you can heal yourself and your family naturally by using essentials oils on your body and in your home.

*****

DEALING WITH DEPRESSION NATURALLY

Dealing with Depression Naturally presents a holistic approach to managing depression with natural antidepressants. You will learn how to treat depression with:

* Aromatherapy

* Art therapy

* Christian Biblical principles

* Chromotherapy

* Diet therapy

* Eco-therapy

* Herbal therapy

* Home decor therapy

* Music therapy

* Phototherapy

* Exercise therapy

* Self-Psychotherapy

* Social therapy

* Talk therapy

* Vitamin therapy

* Writing therapy

*****

CHRISTIAN LIFE COACHING HANDBOOK

Christian Life Coaching Handbook offers a Biblical approach to managing different aspects of life.

You will learn:

* Christian anger management

* Christian conflict resolution

* Christian depression treatment

* Christian goal setting

* Christian marital stress management

* Christian stress management

* How to assert yourself

* How to defeat fear

* How to love yourself

* How to overcome shyness

* How to resist temptation

* How to stop being a people pleaser

*****

CHRISTIAN PERSONAL FINANCE

Christian Personal Finance teaches Biblical principles of money management.

You will learn:

* Christian financial stress management from people who were dealing with money stress like the Acts 3 beggar or credit issues like the widow in second Kings.

* Biblical prosperity principles from wealthy men and women of God like Isaac and the Proverbs 31 woman.

* Bible verses to use as spiritual warfare prayers and as Christian finance affirmations and Christian money meditations.

*****

ANTHOLOGY OF CHRISTIAN BIBLE SERMONS

Anthology of Christian Bible Sermons is a compilation of more than 20 Biblical rhema teachings which include:

* A New Christmas Message

* A New Easter Message

* Are You A Flamboyant Fig Tree Christian?

* Biblical Lessons for Purim from Queen Esther

* Can God Help Me If I Am Surrounded By Enemies?

* How Badly Do You Really Want It?

* Seed Words And The Powerful Tongue

* Spiritual AIDS

* The Three Levels Of Getting Lost

* Why Does God Allow Suffering?

* Your Life Is Your Ministry And Your Storm Is Your Message

* A Perfect God, Imperfect People, and Perfect Plans

* We Are Not Ignorant of His Devices

* How to Prepare for a Dangerous Journey

* Yes, God Can

* How to Serve the Body of Christ

* Conduits of God

* Go Back? Stand Still? Move Forward? Drown?

*****

CHRISTIAN SPIRITUAL WARFARE

Christian Spiritual Warfare teaches you the awesome Bible verses you can use as spiritual warfare prayers, Christian affirmations and in your Christian meditation sessions as you fight your spiritual battles.

You will learn how to fight for the following with Bible verses:

* Marriage * Children * Health

* Christian Faith * Christian Ministry

* Country

* Finances * Job * Business

* Peace of Mind * Restoration * Self Esteem * Self Love

You will also learn how to fight against the following with Bible verses:

* Addiction * Temptation

* Being Single * Infertility

* Opposition * Oppression

* Worry * Fear

* Feelings of Condemnation * Confusion

* Danger * Death * Despair * Discouragement

* Impatience * Insomnia * Laziness * Loneliness

* Poverty * Pride * Sadness

* Vengeance * Weakness

* A Foul Mouth * Lying

*****

DARK SKIN DERMATOLOGY COLOR ATLAS

Dark Skin Dermatology Color Atlas is filled with clear explanations and color photos of skin, hair, and nail diseases affecting people with skin of color or Fitzpatrick skin types IV, V, and VI.

Topics covered include Acne Vulgaris, Alopecia Areata, Anal Warts, Angioedema, Aphthous Ulcers, Atopic Dermatitis, Blastomycosis, Blister Beetle Dermatitis or Nairobi Fly Dermatitis, Cellulitis, Chronic Ulcers, Confetti Hypopigmentation, Cutaneous T Cell Lymphoma, Cutaneous Tuberculosis, Dermatitis Artefacta, Erythema Nodosum,

Exfoliative Erythroderma, Gianotti Crosti Syndrome, Hand Dermatitis, Hemangioma, Herpes Zoster, Ichthyosis, Ingrown Toenails, Irritant Contact Dermatitis, Kaposi Sarcoma, Keloids, Keratoderma Blenorrhagica, Klippel Trenaunay Weber Syndrome, Leishmaniasis, Leprosy, Leukonychia, Lichen Nitidus, Lichen Planus,

Lichenoid Drug Eruption, Linear Epidermal Nevus, Linear IgA Dermatosis (LAD), Lipodermatosclerosis, Lymphangioma Circumscriptum, Miliaria, Molluscum Contagiosum, Neurofibromatosis, Nickel Dermatitis, Onychomadesis, Onychomycosis, Palmoplantar Eccrine Hidradenitis, Papular Pruritic Eruption (PPE), Paronychia, Pellagra, Pemphigus Foliaceous,

Pemphigus Vulgaris, Piebaldism, Pityriasis Rosea, Pityriasis Rubra Pilaris, Plantar Hyperkeratosis, Plantar Warts, Poikiloderma, Postinflammatory Hyperpigmentation and Hypopigmentation, Post Topical Steroids Hypopigmentation, Psoriasis, Pyogenic Granuloma or Lobular Capillary Hemangioma, Scabies, Seborrheic Dermatitis, Steven Johnson Syndrome (SJS) and Toxic Epidermal Necrolysis (TEN),

Sunburn, Systemic Sclerosis, Tinea Capitis, Tinea Pedis, Tinea Versicolor, Traction Alopecia, Urticaria, Vasculitis, Vitiligo, and Xanthelasma.

*****